The Ultimate Guide to Balcony Gardening for Beginner's

Growing Your Own Oasis

in 2023

By

Jean Burnett

Table of Content

INTRODUCTION

Are you tired of staring out at a barren concrete slab every time you step onto your balcony? Do you long for a lush and vibrant oasis, a place where you can escape the chaos of the city and connect with nature? If so, this book is for you.

In "The Ultimate Guide to Balcony Gardening for Beginner's," we'll show you how to transform your small outdoor space into a thriving garden, bursting with color and life. Whether you're a complete beginner or an experienced gardener, this book is packed with practical tips, step-by-step guides, and beautiful photos to inspire and guide you.

From choosing the right plants for your balcony's conditions to creating a stunning vertical garden, this book covers everything you need to know to create your own urban oasis. You'll learn how to use every inch of your balcony space, whether you have a tiny apartment balcony or a sprawling rooftop terrace.

But this book is about more than just gardening. It's about creating a space that nourishes your soul and connects you with the natural world. It's about finding peace and serenity in the midst of the hustle and bustle of city life. So, join us on this journey and let's grow our own oasis together."

Do you dream of having your own garden, but think it's impossible because you live in an apartment or have a small balcony? Think again. With "The Ultimate Guide to Balcony Gardening," you can create a beautiful garden oasis right outside your door.

In this book, we'll guide you step-by-step through the process of designing, planting, and maintaining a thriving balcony garden. You'll learn how to select the right plants for your space, how to create a successful container garden, and how to care for your plants to ensure they thrive.

But this book is more than just a how-to guide. It's an invitation to slow down and connect with nature, even in the midst of a busy city. It's a reminder that you don't need a large yard or a green thumb to create a beautiful and rewarding garden.

Through stunning photos and inspiring stories, we'll show you how a small balcony can be transformed into a lush and vibrant garden, a place to relax, recharge, and reconnect with the natural world. So if you're ready to take your balcony to the next level, let's get started."

CHAPTER ONE
Getting Started with Balcony Gardening

If you've never gardened before or have only grown plants in a yard, you may be wondering how to get started with balcony gardening. This chapter will provide an overview of the benefits of balcony gardening, assess your balcony space, and provide an overview of the basic tools and equipment needed for balcony gardening.

1.1 The Benefits of Balcony Gardening

Balcony gardening offers a number of benefits, including:

Access to fresh herbs, fruits, and vegetables: When you grow your own food, you know exactly what you're eating and can enjoy fresh, organic produce right from your balcony.

Improved air quality: Plants absorb carbon dioxide and release oxygen, which can help purify the air around your home.

Reduced stress: Gardening has been shown to reduce stress and promote relaxation.

Increased biodiversity: Balcony gardens can help support local pollinators, such as bees and butterflies.

1.2 Assessing Your Balcony Space

Before you start planting, it's important to assess your balcony space. Consider the following factors:

Size: How much space do you have to work with? You'll want to choose plants that fit comfortably within your balcony space.

Exposure: What direction does your balcony face? How much sun does it get? Different plants have different light requirements, so it's important to choose plants that will thrive in your balcony's conditions.

Accessibility: How easy is it to access your balcony? If you live on an upper floor, you'll need to consider how you'll transport soil, plants, and equipment up and down the stairs or elevator.

1.3 Choosing Containers and Soil

One of the most important considerations for balcony gardening is choosing the right containers and soil. Consider the following factors:

Size: Choose containers that are appropriate for the size of your plants. Larger plants will need larger containers to accommodate their roots.

Drainage: Make sure your containers have drainage holes to prevent water from pooling and causing root rot.

Material: Choose containers made from materials that will withstand the elements, such as plastic, metal, or ceramic.

Soil: Choose a high-quality potting mix that is appropriate for your plants' needs. Look for mixes that are designed for container gardening and provide good drainage.

1.4 Basic Tools and Equipment

To get started with balcony gardening, you'll need a few basic tools and equipment, including:

Hand trowel and fork: These tools are essential for planting and maintaining your balcony garden.

Watering can or hose: You'll need a way to water your plants regularly.

Pruning shears: These are used to trim dead or damaged plant material.

Fertilizer: Choose a high-quality fertilizer that is appropriate for your plants' needs.

Pesticides: Insects and diseases can be a problem for balcony gardens, so it's important to have an appropriate pesticide on hand.

By assessing your balcony space, choosing the right containers and soil, and gathering the basic tools and equipment, you'll be well on your way to creating a thriving balcony garden.

1.5 Assessing Your Balcony Space: Size

When assessing the size of your balcony space, it's important to consider both the amount of floor space available and the vertical space you have to work with. Balcony gardens can make use of all three dimensions, so don't forget to look up as well as out.

For example, you can hang plants from the balcony ceiling or walls using hanging baskets or planters. You can also use a trellis or other support to create a vertical garden, allowing you to grow climbing plants like beans, cucumbers, and tomatoes.

When choosing plants for a small balcony, consider varieties that are compact or have a trailing habit, such as cherry tomatoes or trailing petunias. You can also use space-saving techniques like growing plants in a tiered planter or creating a vertical herb garden using a repurposed pallet.

1.6 Assessing Your Balcony Space: Exposure

The amount of sun or shade your balcony receives will have a big impact on the plants you can grow. Most plants need at least six hours of direct sunlight per day to thrive, although there are some varieties that can tolerate partial or full shade. If your balcony faces north or east, it may receive less direct sunlight and be cooler than a balcony that faces south or west. In this case, you may need to choose plants that are shade-tolerant or prefer cooler temperatures.

On the other hand, if your balcony is in a hot, sunny location, you may need to choose plants that are drought-tolerant and can withstand high temperatures.

1.7 Choosing Containers and Soil

Choosing the right containers and soil is crucial for balcony gardening success. Here are some tips to help you get started: Choose containers that are large enough to accommodate your plants' root systems. If you're growing vegetables or other large plants, you may need containers that are at least 12 inches deep.

Make sure your containers have drainage holes to prevent water from pooling and causing root rot.

Consider the material of your containers. Plastic containers are lightweight and easy to move, while ceramic or metal containers can add a decorative touch to your balcony garden. Choose a high-quality potting mix that is appropriate for your plants' needs. Look for mixes that are designed for container gardening and provide good drainage.

1.8 Basic Tools and Equipment

To get started with balcony gardening, you'll need a few basic tools and equipment. Here are some of the essentials:

Hand trowel and fork: These tools are essential for planting and maintaining your balcony garden. Choose tools that are comfortable to use and made of sturdy materials.

Watering can or hose: You'll need a way to water your plants regularly. If you have a large balcony garden, a hose may be more practical.

Pruning shears: These are used to trim dead or damaged plant material. Make sure you keep your shears sharp to prevent damaging your plants.

Fertilizer: Choose a high-quality fertilizer that is appropriate for your plants' needs. Different plants have different nutrient requirements, so make sure you choose a fertilizer that is appropriate for your specific plants.

Pesticides: Insects and diseases can be a problem for balcony gardens, so it's important to have an appropriate pesticide on hand. Choose a pesticide that is safe for use on edible plants and follow the instructions carefully.

By assessing your balcony space, choosing the right containers and soil, and gathering the basic tools and equipment, you'll be well on your way to creating a thriving balcony garden. With a little bit of planning and preparation, you can enjoy fresh herbs, vegetables, and flowers right outside your door.

CHAPTER TWO
Choosing Plants for Your Balcony Garden

Now that you've assessed your balcony space and gathered the necessary tools and equipment, it's time to choose the plants for your balcony garden. There are a few key factors to consider when choosing plants, including the amount of sunlight your balcony receives, the size of your containers, and the amount of maintenance you're willing to put in.

2.1 Sunlight Requirements

As mentioned in Chapter 1, the amount of sunlight your balcony receives will have a big impact on the plants you can grow. Most plants need at least six hours of direct sunlight per day to thrive, although there are some varieties that can tolerate partial or full shade.

If your balcony faces north or east and receives less direct sunlight, you may need to choose plants that are shade-tolerant or prefer cooler temperatures. Examples of shade-tolerant plants include ferns, hosts, and impatiens.

On the other hand, if your balcony is in a hot, sunny location, you may need to choose plants that are drought-tolerant and can withstand high temperatures. Examples of drought-tolerant plants include succulents, lavender, and rosemary.

2.2 Container Size

The size of your containers will also affect the plants you can grow. Generally, the larger the container, the more soil it can hold, which means more room for the plant's roots to grow.

If you're growing vegetables or other large plants, you may need containers that are at least 12 inches deep. For herbs or smaller plants, containers that are 6-8 inches deep may be sufficient.

It's also important to consider the width of your containers. Plants that have a trailing habit, such as petunias or ivy, will require wider containers to allow for their growth.

2.3 Maintenance Requirements

The amount of maintenance you're willing to put in will also affect the plants you choose for your balcony garden. Some plants require more care than others, so consider how much time and effort you're willing to dedicate to your garden.

For example, herbs like basil and parsley are relatively easy to care for and require minimal maintenance, while tomatoes and peppers may require more attention, such as staking or pruning.

2.4 Choosing Plants for Aesthetic Appeal

In addition to considering the practical factors of sunlight and maintenance, it's also important to choose plants that you find visually appealing. Consider the colors and textures of the plants, as well as how they will look in combination with other plants.

For example, a mix of trailing ivy and brightly colored petunias can create a beautiful and eye-catching display. Mixing in herbs like thyme or rosemary can also add interesting textures and scents to your balcony garden.

2.5 Choosing Plants for Food Production

If you're interested in growing your own food, there are plenty of options for balcony gardening. Many vegetables can be grown in containers, including tomatoes, peppers, cucumbers, and beans.

Herbs are also a great option for balcony gardens, as they are often small and require minimal maintenance. Basil, parsley, and chives are all great options for beginners.

It's important to note that some plants may require additional support or staking as they grow, so be sure to research the specific needs of the plants you choose.

Overall, there are many factors to consider when choosing plants for your balcony garden, including sunlight requirements, container size, maintenance requirements, aesthetic appeal, and food production potential. By taking the time to carefully choose your plants, you can create a beautiful and thriving balcony garden that meets your needs and preferences.

2.6 Consider Companion Planting

Another factor to consider when choosing plants for your balcony garden is companion planting. Companion planting is the practice of planting certain species of plants together in order to benefit one or both of the plants.

For example, planting marigolds with your vegetables can help to deter pests, while planting herbs like mint or lavender near your vegetables can help to repel insects.

Companion planting can also help to improve soil health by adding nutrients to the soil or improving drainage. For example, planting legumes like beans or peas can help to fix nitrogen in the soil, which is beneficial for other plants.

2.7 Research Plant Requirements

Before you choose your plants, it's important to research their specific requirements in terms of soil, water, and nutrients. Some plants may require more frequent watering or fertilizing than others, so it's important to understand their needs in order to ensure their success.

It's also important to choose plants that are suited to your climate and growing zone. Different plants have different temperature and humidity requirements, so be sure to choose plants that are well-suited to your local climate.

2.8 Start Small and Experiment

If you're new to balcony gardening, it's a good idea to start small and experiment with a few plants before investing in a larger garden. This will allow you to learn the basics of balcony gardening and get a feel for what works best in your space.

You may also want to consider starting with easy-to-grow plants like herbs or lettuces, which require minimal maintenance and can be harvested relatively quickly.

As you gain experience and confidence, you can start to expand your garden and try new plants and techniques.

2.9 Common Plants for Balcony Gardens

Here are some common plants that are well-suited to balcony gardens:

Herbs: Basil, parsley, chives, thyme, rosemary, oregano, mint

Vegetables: Tomatoes, peppers, lettuce, spinach, cucumbers, beans, peas

Flowers: Petunias, geraniums, impatiens, marigolds, pansies, snapdragons, daisies

Keep in mind that this is just a starting point, and there are many other plants that can thrive in balcony gardens. Be sure to do your research and choose plants that are well-suited to your specific balcony environment and your own personal preferences.

2.10 Container Gardening Techniques

When it comes to balcony gardening, container gardening is the most popular technique. Container gardening involves planting your plants in containers or pots instead of directly in the ground.

There are a variety of container options available, including traditional terracotta pots, hanging baskets, and window boxes. When choosing containers for your balcony garden, it's important to consider the size of your plants and their root systems.

Some plants require deeper pots, while others can thrive in shallow containers. You'll also need to consider the drainage of your containers, as plants can quickly become waterlogged and suffer from root rot if the soil is constantly wet.

2.11 Soil and Fertilizers

Choosing the right soil and fertilizers is crucial for the success of your balcony garden. When it comes to soil, it's important to choose a high-quality potting mix that is specifically formulated for container gardening.

These mixes are typically lighter and more porous than traditional garden soil, allowing for better drainage and aeration. You can also add amendments like perlite or vermiculite to improve drainage and water retention.

When it comes to fertilizers, there are a variety of options available, including organic and synthetic fertilizers. Organic fertilizers like compost or worm castings are a great choice for balcony gardens, as they help to improve soil health and promote healthy plant growth.

2.12 Watering and Maintenance

Proper watering and maintenance are essential for the success of your balcony garden. Most plants require consistent watering, but the frequency and amount of water needed can vary depending on the plant and the weather.

As a general rule, it's better to underwater than overwater your plants, as too much water can lead to root rot and other issues. You can use a moisture meter or simply stick your finger into the soil to determine whether your plants need watering.

In addition to watering, you'll also need to maintain your balcony garden by pruning, deadheading, and removing any dead or diseased plant material. Regular maintenance will help to keep your plants healthy and thriving.

By following these tips and techniques, you can create a beautiful and thriving balcony garden that will provide you with fresh herbs, vegetables, and flowers all season long.'

CHAPTER THREE
Maximizing Your Balcony Garden Space

One of the biggest challenges of balcony gardening is the limited space available. However, with some creativity and strategic planning, you can maximize your balcony garden space and create a beautiful and productive garden.

3.1 Vertical Gardening

Vertical gardening is a technique that involves growing plants vertically, rather than horizontally. This can be achieved by using trellises, hanging baskets, or stacked planters.

Vertical gardening allows you to make the most of your vertical space and grow more plants in a smaller area. It's also a great way to add visual interest and texture to your balcony garden.

When choosing plants for vertical gardening, consider their growth habit and how they will respond to being trained vertically. Climbing plants like cucumbers, tomatoes, and beans are well-suited to vertical gardening, as are trailing plants like petunias and nasturtiums.

3.2 Container Grouping

Another way to maximize your balcony garden space is by grouping containers together. By clustering pots and containers, you can create a lusher and more cohesive look, while also maximizing your planting space.

When grouping containers, consider the size and shape of your pots, as well as the size and growth habit of your plants. You'll also need to consider how much sun and shade each plant requires, and make sure to group plants with similar light requirements together.

You can also experiment with different container heights and textures to create a more dynamic and visually interesting display.

3.3 Edible Landscaping

Edible landscaping is a technique that involves incorporating edible plants into your landscape design. This can be a great way to maximize your balcony garden space while also providing you with fresh and nutritious produce.

When planning your edible landscape, consider the size and growth habit of your plants, as well as their aesthetic appeal. You'll also need to consider the amount of sunlight and water each plant requires, and make sure to group plants with similar needs together.

Some edible plants that are well-suited to balcony gardening include herbs like basil and parsley, salad greens like lettuce and spinach, and compact vegetables like cherry tomatoes and peppers.

3.4 Creative Planters

Finally, one of the most effective ways to maximize your balcony garden space is by using creative and unconventional planters. There are a variety of container options available, from repurposed items like old boots and tin cans to specialized planters like strawberry towers and vertical gardens.

When choosing creative planters, consider the size and shape of your balcony, as well as your personal style and aesthetic preferences. You can also experiment with different materials like wood, metal, and plastic to create a unique and personalized look.

By using these techniques and strategies, you can maximize your balcony garden space and create a beautiful and productive garden that will provide you with fresh herbs, vegetables, and flowers all season long.

3.5 Companion Planting

Companion planting is a technique that involves planting different species of plants together that benefit each other in some way. This can include plants that attract beneficial insects or repel pests, plants that provide shade or support to other plants, or plants that share nutrients and resources.

Companion planting can be especially helpful in small balcony gardens, where space is limited and plants are in close proximity to each other. Some popular companion plants include marigolds, which repel pests like aphids and attract beneficial insects like ladybugs, and basil, which improves the flavor and growth of tomatoes.

When planning your balcony garden, consider incorporating companion planting techniques to create a more sustainable and self-sufficient garden.

3.6 Vertical Hydroponics

Hydroponics is a soil-free method of growing plants that uses nutrient-rich water to support plant growth. This can be an effective way to maximize your balcony garden space and grow a wide variety of plants in a small area.

Vertical hydroponics is a technique that involves stacking hydroponic systems vertically to create a more efficient and space-saving growing system. This can include using vertical towers or racks to grow plants, or hanging hydroponic baskets from a trellis or railing.

When using hydroponics in your balcony garden, be sure to choose plants that are well-suited to this growing method, and follow the specific instructions for your hydroponic system.

By incorporating these techniques and strategies into your balcony gardening plan, you can maximize your space and create a beautiful and productive garden that provides you with fresh and healthy produce all season long.

3.7 Microgreens and Sprouts

Microgreens and sprouts are two popular options for growing nutritious and delicious greens in a small space. Microgreens are young plants that are harvested when they are only a few inches tall, while sprouts are the germinated seeds of plants that are eaten when they are still in their early stages of growth.

Both microgreens and sprouts are packed with nutrients and are easy to grow indoors or on a balcony. They can be grown in small containers or trays, and require minimal space and maintenance.

When growing microgreens or sprouts, be sure to choose seeds that are well-suited to your growing conditions and follow the specific instructions for your chosen method.

3.8 Creative Use of Space

Finally, one of the keys to maximizing your balcony garden space is to get creative with your use of space. This can include using window boxes, hanging planters, or shelves to add more planting space, or incorporating vertical elements like trellises and ladders to create more growing opportunities.

You can also experiment with different growing methods like aquaponics, which combines hydroponics with aquaculture to create a closed-loop system that recycles nutrients and water.

By getting creative with your use of space and experimenting with different growing techniques, you can create a beautiful and productive balcony garden that maximizes your space and provides you with fresh and healthy produce all season long.

CHAPTER FOUR

Maintaining Your Balcony Garden

Now that you have set up your balcony garden and have plants growing, it is important to maintain it properly to ensure a healthy and bountiful harvest. In this chapter, we will explore some important tips and techniques for maintaining your balcony garden.

4.1 Watering Your Plants

Watering your plants is one of the most important aspects of maintaining a healthy balcony garden. It is essential to keep your plants hydrated, but over-watering can lead to root rot and other problems.

The frequency and amount of watering will depend on a variety of factors, including the type of plants, the size of containers, and the weather conditions. As a general rule, it is better to water deeply and less frequently, rather than lightly and frequently.

To determine when to water, stick your finger into the soil to see if it feels dry. If it is dry to the touch, it is time to water. You can also invest in a moisture meter to help you monitor the moisture levels of your soil.

4.2 Fertilizing Your Plants

In addition to water, your plants will need nutrients to grow healthy and strong. Fertilizing your plants is a crucial part of balcony garden maintenance.

There are many different types of fertilizers available, including organic and synthetic options. Organic fertilizers are made from natural sources like compost, manure, or bone meal, and are typically more sustainable and environmentally friendly.

When fertilizing your plants, be sure to follow the instructions carefully and avoid over-fertilizing, as this can lead to fertilizer burn and other problems.

4.3 Pest Control

Pests like aphids, mites, and other insects can wreak havoc on your balcony garden. There are many different methods for controlling pests, including natural options like insecticidal soaps, neem oil, or diatomaceous earth, as well as synthetic options like pesticides.

It is important to choose a pest control method that is safe for your plants and the environment, and to follow the instructions carefully to avoid overuse or misuse.

4.4 Pruning and Harvesting

Pruning and harvesting your plants is an important part of maintaining a healthy balcony garden. Regular pruning can help to promote healthy growth and prevent disease, while harvesting your crops at the right time can help to ensure optimal flavor and nutrition.

When pruning, be sure to use sharp and clean tools to avoid damaging your plants, and to follow the specific instructions for your plants.

When harvesting your crops, be sure to pick them at the right time to ensure maximum flavor and nutrition. Different plants will have different harvesting requirements, so be sure to do your research before picking your crops.

4.5 Winterizing Your Balcony Garden

Finally, if you live in a colder climate, it is important to winterize your balcony garden to protect your plants from the harsh winter weather. This can include bringing your plants indoors, covering them with frost blankets or other protective covers, or simply removing them and starting fresh in the spring.

By following these important tips and techniques for maintaining your balcony garden, you can ensure a healthy and bountiful harvest all season long.

4.6 Dealing with Weather Challenges

While balcony gardening can be a rewarding and enjoyable experience, it can also come with some challenges, particularly when it comes to weather. Hot, dry weather can quickly dry out soil and damage plants, while wet weather can lead to fungal growth and other problems.

To deal with these challenges, it is important to stay vigilant and take steps to protect your plants. This can include using shade cloth or umbrellas to protect plants from direct sunlight during hot weather, or using a fan or misting system to cool down plants.

In wet weather, it is important to avoid overwatering and to ensure proper drainage to prevent waterlogged soil. You can also use organic fungicides or other methods to control fungal growth and other problems.

4.7 Keeping a Garden Journal

One useful tool for maintaining a balcony garden is to keep a garden journal. This can help you keep track of important information like planting dates, watering and fertilizing schedules, and pest control methods.

A garden journal can also help you identify patterns and trends in your garden, and can serve as a useful reference tool for future balcony gardening endeavors.

4.8 Staying Motivated

Finally, it is important to stay motivated and inspired when maintaining your balcony garden. One way to do this is to set goals and track your progress, whether it is growing a specific crop or simply improving your gardening skills.

You can also seek out resources like gardening blogs, forums, or social media groups to connect with other gardeners and share tips and advice. By staying motivated and inspired, you can continue to enjoy the many benefits of balcony gardening for years to come.

4.9 Common Pests and Diseases

Despite our best efforts, sometimes pests and diseases can still invade our balcony gardens. Some common pests include aphids, spider mites, and whiteflies, while common diseases include powdery mildew and leaf spot.

To prevent and control pests and diseases, it is important to practice good garden hygiene, such as regularly removing dead or diseased plant material and keeping the area clean. You can also use natural methods like companion planting or organic pesticides, or consult with a gardening expert for more specific advice.

4.10 Harvesting and Preserving

One of the most satisfying aspects of balcony gardening is harvesting and enjoying your own fresh produce. When it comes to harvesting, it is important to do so at the right time and in the right way, whether it is picking fruits and vegetables when they are ripe or harvesting herbs before they flower.

To preserve your harvest, there are several methods you can use, such as freezing, canning, or drying. This can help you enjoy your produce even after the growing season is over.

CHAPTER FIVE
Advanced Techniques and Tips for Balcony Gardening

In the previous chapters, we covered the basics of balcony gardening, including selecting the right plants, soil, containers, and more. In this chapter, we will explore some advanced techniques and tips that can help take your balcony garden to the next level.

5.1 Vertical Gardening

One popular technique for maximizing space in a small balcony garden is vertical gardening. This involves growing plants vertically, either by using trellises, hanging baskets, or vertical planters.

Vertical gardening not only saves space but can also create a visually striking garden that adds interest and texture to your balcony. It can also help to provide shade and privacy, as well as reduce noise and air pollution.

5.2 Hydroponics

Hydroponics is a technique of growing plants without soil, using nutrient-rich water instead. This technique can be especially useful for balcony gardening, as it allows you to grow more plants in less space and with less water.

To set up a hydroponic system, you will need a container, a water pump, a timer, and a nutrient solution. There are many types of hydroponic systems, including deep water culture, nutrient film technique, and drip irrigation.

While hydroponics can be more expensive and complex than traditional soil-based gardening, it can also yield faster growth and higher yields, making it a worthwhile investment for serious balcony gardeners.

5.3 Green Roofs

Another advanced technique for balcony gardening is green roofs, which involve growing plants on the roof of your building. Green roofs not only provide an attractive garden space but also offer several environmental benefits, such as reducing urban heat island effects and improving air quality.

To create a green roof, you will need a waterproof membrane, drainage layer, growing medium, and plants. There are many types of green roof systems, including intensive and extensive systems, which vary in their soil depth and plant choices.

While creating a green roof can be a complex and expensive undertaking, it can also provide a beautiful and sustainable garden space that adds value to your home and community.

5.4 Advanced Plant Care Techniques

As your balcony garden grows, you may encounter new challenges and opportunities for advanced plant care techniques. These can include things like pruning, grafting, and propagation.

Pruning involves cutting back plants to encourage new growth and improve their shape and health. Grafting involves joining two plants together to create a new hybrid plant, while propagation involves growing new plants from cuttings or seeds.

By mastering these techniques, you can create a more diverse and resilient balcony garden that yields higher yields and greater satisfaction.

5.6 Seasonal Gardening

One way to keep your balcony garden thriving year-round is to practice seasonal gardening. This involves planting different crops at different times of the year, depending on the season and weather conditions.

For example, in the spring, you may plant cool-season crops like lettuce, peas, and spinach, while in the summer, you may plant warm-season crops like tomatoes, peppers, and eggplants. In the fall, you may plant cool-season crops again, such as kale, broccoli, and cauliflower.

By practicing seasonal gardening, you can ensure that your balcony garden is always filled with fresh and delicious produce, no matter what time of the year it is.

5.7 Companion Planting

Companion planting is another advanced technique that can improve the health and productivity of your balcony garden.

This involves planting different crops together that have complementary needs and benefits.

For example, planting basil with tomatoes can help repel pests and improve the flavor of the tomatoes, while planting marigolds with beans can help repel harmful nematodes in the soil.

By practicing companion planting, you can create a more diverse and resilient garden that is better able to resist pests and diseases and produce higher yields.

5.8 Using Artificial Lighting

In some cases, your balcony garden may not receive enough natural sunlight to grow certain plants, especially during the winter months. In these cases, you can use artificial lighting, such as grow lights, to supplement the natural light and provide your plants with the necessary light spectrum for growth.

When using grow lights, it is important to choose the right type of light for your plants, as different types of plants require different light spectra. It is also important to position the lights at the right distance from the plants to avoid burning or damaging them.

By using artificial lighting, you can expand the range of plants you can grow in your balcony garden and ensure that they receive the necessary light for healthy growth.

5.10 Maintaining Your Balcony Garden

No matter how advanced your techniques and strategies are, maintaining your balcony garden is essential for its success. This includes regular watering, fertilizing, pruning, and pest management.

Watering: Make sure to water your plants regularly, but be careful not to overwater them. The frequency and amount of watering may vary depending on the type of plant and weather conditions.

Fertilizing: Your plants will also need regular fertilization to maintain healthy growth and productivity. You can use organic fertilizers or create your own compost for this purpose.

Pruning: Pruning your plants is important for maintaining their shape and preventing overgrowth. It can also improve air circulation and reduce the risk of diseases.

Pest Management: Pest management is crucial for protecting your plants from harmful insects and diseases. You can use natural pest control methods or organic pesticides for this purpose.

5.11 Troubleshooting Common Problems

Despite your best efforts, you may still encounter common problems in your balcony garden, such as pests, diseases, or environmental factors. It is important to identify these problems early and take appropriate action to prevent further damage.

Some common problems and their solutions include:

Pests: Use natural pest control methods, such as companion planting or insect-repelling herbs, or organic pesticides to control pests.

Diseases: Practice good hygiene and sanitation, such as removing infected plants and disinfecting your tools. You can also use organic fungicides to control fungal diseases.

Environmental Factors: Adjust your watering and fertilizing schedule according to weather conditions. Provide shade or artificial lighting as needed to protect your plants from extreme temperatures.

5.12 Final Thoughts

Balcony gardening is a rewarding and enjoyable hobby that can bring fresh produce and beauty to your home. By using advanced techniques and strategies, you can take your balcony garden to the next level and create a thriving and sustainable oasis in the midst of the city.

Remember to start small, choose the right plants for your space and climate, and maintain good gardening practices to ensure the success of your balcony garden. With patience, dedication, and a little creativity, you can grow a beautiful and productive garden on your balcony.

CHAPTER SIX

Going Beyond the Basics: Advanced Techniques for Balcony Gardening

Congratulations! By now, you have become an expert in the basics of balcony gardening. You have learned how to choose the right plants, prepare your space, and care for your plants. But there are many more advanced techniques you can use to take your balcony garden to the next level. In this chapter, we will explore some of these techniques.

6.1 Intensive Gardening Techniques

Intensive gardening techniques involve maximizing plant density and productivity in a limited space. Some common techniques include:

Vertical Gardening: Vertical gardening involves growing plants vertically, either on trellises or using specialized containers. This allows you to make the most of your limited space and create a lush, green wall.

Square Foot Gardening: Square foot gardening involves dividing your space into small, square sections and planting a different crop in each section. This allows you to maximize productivity and reduce waste.

Companion Planting: Companion planting involves planting two or more crops together that complement each other. For example, planting marigolds alongside tomatoes can help repel pests and improve soil health.

6.2 Hydroponics

Hydroponics is a method of growing plants without soil, using nutrient-rich water instead. Hydroponics can be a great option for balcony gardens, as it allows you to grow plants vertically and in small spaces. Some common hydroponic systems include:

Drip Systems: Drip systems involve delivering nutrient-rich water directly to the roots of the plants, either through a timer or manually.

Nutrient Film Technique: Nutrient film technique involves creating a shallow, constantly flowing stream of nutrient-rich water over the roots of the plants.

Wick Systems: Wick systems involve using a wick to draw water from a reservoir to the plants' roots.

6.3 Advanced Lighting Techniques

Lighting is crucial for plant growth and productivity, especially in indoor balcony gardens. Some advanced lighting techniques include:

LED Grow Lights: LED grow lights provide full-spectrum light that mimics natural sunlight and can be adjusted to suit different plants' needs.

Reflectors: Reflectors can help maximize the amount of light your plants receive by reflecting it back onto the plants.

6.4 Integrated Pest Management

Integrated pest management (IPM) is a holistic approach to pest control that involves using multiple strategies to prevent and control pests. Some common IPM techniques include:

Biological Control: Biological control involves using natural enemies of pests, such as ladybugs or nematodes, to control them.

Cultural Control: Cultural control involves modifying your gardening practices to reduce pest problems, such as rotating crops or pruning plants.

Chemical Control: Chemical control involves using pesticides as a last resort and only when necessary.

6.5 Advanced Soil Management

Soil management is crucial for healthy plant growth and productivity. Some advanced soil management techniques include:

Soil Testing: Soil testing involves testing your soil for pH, nutrient levels, and other factors to determine if it needs amending.

Composting: Composting involves creating a nutrient-rich soil amendment from organic matter, such as food scraps and yard waste.

Mulching: Mulching involves adding a layer of organic material, such as leaves or straw, to the soil's surface to retain moisture and suppress weeds.

6.6 Dealing with Common Challenges

Even with the best techniques and practices, balcony gardening can still present its own set of challenges. Here are some common issues you may face and how to overcome them:

Pests: Pests can wreak havoc on your plants, so it's important to identify and control them early. Some common pests in balcony gardens include aphids, spider mites, and whiteflies. Use integrated pest management techniques to control them.

Limited Space: Limited space is one of the biggest challenges of balcony gardening. To maximize space, use vertical gardening techniques, choose compact plants, and use hanging baskets and containers.

Sun Exposure: Balconies can be exposed to harsh sunlight or shade, depending on their orientation. Choose plants that can tolerate your balcony's sun exposure and use shade cloth or umbrellas to protect them.

Soil Quality: Balcony gardens often use potting soil, which can become depleted of nutrients over time. Use compost and other soil amendments to improve soil quality.

6.7 Further Resources

If you want to learn more about advanced techniques for balcony gardening, there are many resources available to you. Here are a few recommendations:

Vertical Gardening: Vertical gardening is an effective way to maximize space in your balcony garden. The book "The Vertical Garden: From Nature to the City" by Patrick Blanc is a great resource for learning about this technique.

Hydroponics: Hydroponics is a soil-free method of growing plants using nutrient-rich water. "Hydroponic Basics" by George F. Van Patten is an excellent resource for beginners.

Lighting: If you are interested in using artificial lighting to grow plants in your balcony garden, "Indoor Gardening: The Ultimate Guide to Growing Vegetables, Fruits, and Herbs Indoors" by Emily Parker is a great resource.

Integrated Pest Management: "Integrated Pest Management for Home Gardeners and Landscape Professionals" by University of California Agriculture and Natural Resources is an excellent resource for learning how to control pests in a sustainable and environmentally friendly way.

Soil Quality: "The Vegetable Gardener's Bible" by Edward C. Smith is a great resource for learning about soil health and soil improvement techniques.

These resources can provide you with more in-depth information on specific topics related to balcony gardening. By using these resources in conjunction with the techniques outlined in this chapter, you can take your balcony garden to the next level.

6.8 Final Thoughts

By using these advanced techniques, you can take your balcony garden to the next level and create a thriving and sustainable oasis in the midst of the city. Remember to start small and experiment with different techniques to find what works best for your space, climate, and gardening style. With patience, dedication, and a little creativity, you can grow a beautiful and productive garden on your balcony.

CONCLUSION

Balcony Gardening for Beginners: is the definitive guide for anyone looking to create a beautiful and sustainable garden on their balcony. Whether you're a seasoned gardener or a complete beginner, this book will provide you with the knowledge, skills, and inspiration to create a thriving garden that reflects your unique style and personality.

With detailed explanations and step-by-step instructions, this book covers everything from plant selection and soil quality to lighting and pest management. You'll explore a range of innovative techniques, including hydroponics, vertical gardening, and organic pest control. And with beautiful photographs and engaging prose, this book is as visually stunning as it is informative.

But it's not just about the practicalities of gardening. This book is also a celebration of the joy and satisfaction that comes from connecting with nature and nurturing living things. Whether you're looking to grow your own food, create a peaceful oasis in the midst of the city, or simply enjoy the beauty of nature, this book will empower you to create a garden that meets your unique needs and desires.

So, whether you're looking to improve your mental and emotional wellbeing, reduce your environmental impact, or simply have fun, "Balcony Gardening for Beginners: Advanced Techniques and Practices" is the perfect guide for you. With this book in hand, you'll have everything you need to create a beautiful, sustainable garden that will bring joy and inspiration for years to come.

www.ingramcontent.com/pod-product-compliance
Lightning Source LLC
Chambersburg PA
CBHW061534250726